COOKING WITH CANCER FIGHTING FOODS

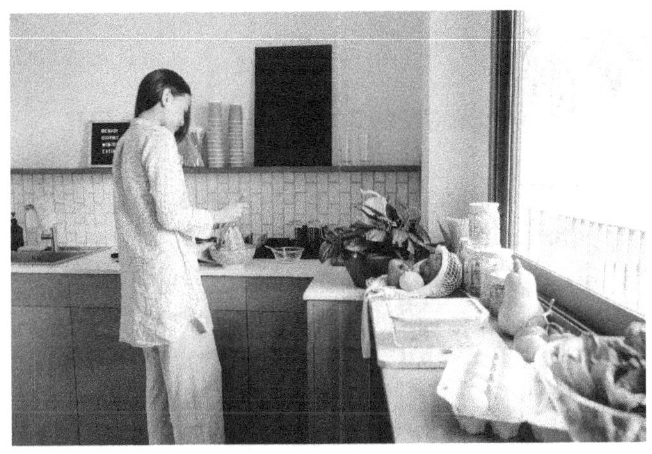

A diet cookbook for cancer prevention, treatment and recovery

HILDA PARKER

TABLE OF CONTENT

INTRODUCTION

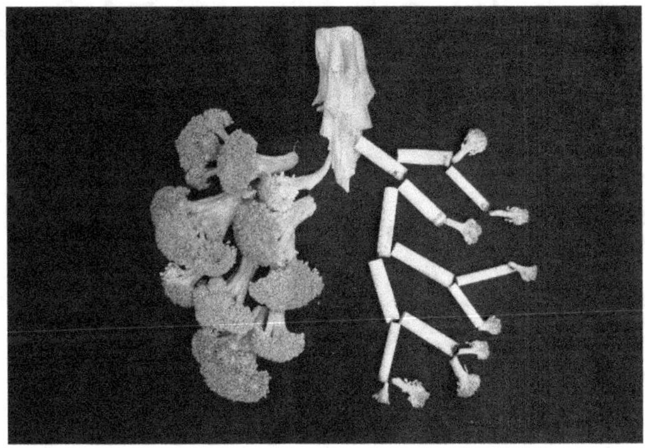

In an era where health-conscious living takes centre stage, and the pursuit of well-being transcends mere trends, the intersection of science and gastronomy becomes a beacon of hope. The "Foods That Beat Cancer Cookbook" emerges as a comprehensive guide, inviting readers to embark on a culinary journey that intertwines the pleasures of eating with the potential for prevention and healing.

Cancer, an affliction that has touched countless lives, continues to be a subject of profound concern. As research into the connections between diet and disease advances, the power of food in promoting health gains prominence. Drawing from the latest findings in nutritional science, this cookbook seamlessly marries flavours and nutrients in dishes designed not only to tantalise the palate but also to fortify the body.

Within the pages of this cookbook, the art of cooking converges with the science of nourishment. Each recipe is meticulously crafted to include ingredients rich in antioxidants, phytochemicals, and other bioactive compounds known for their potential to combat the development and progression of cancer cells. From vibrant salads bursting with colourful vegetables to sumptuous main courses featuring lean proteins and delectable desserts, every dish is an invitation to savour not just the taste, but the promise of vitality.

However, this book isn't merely a collection of recipes. It's a source of empowerment and education. Alongside each culinary creation, you'll find insights into the nutritional benefits of key ingredients, explanations of the scientific concepts that underpin their cancer-fighting potential, and practical tips for integrating these foods into your everyday life. It's a holistic approach that extends beyond the kitchen, fostering an understanding of the profound impact our dietary choices can have on our overall health.

Whether you're someone seeking ways to proactively reduce the risk of cancer, a caregiver supporting a loved one's wellness journey, or an individual navigating life post-diagnosis, the "Foods That Beat Cancer Cookbook" is your steadfast companion. It's a testament to the idea that food isn't just sustenance; it's a potent ally in the fight for health and vitality. So, step into your kitchen with purpose, armed with the knowledge that each meal can be a small but meaningful stride towards a life of wellness.

UNDERSTANDING CANCER AND DIET

Cancer is a complicated category of diseases characterised by uncontrolled growth and cell growth. While the development of cancer is influenced by a combination of genetic, environmental, and lifestyle factors, emerging research suggests that diet plays a significant role in both the prevention and management of cancer. Certain foods are believed to have properties that can help fight cancer, thanks to their abundance of beneficial compounds such as antioxidants, phytochemicals, vitamins, and minerals. Here, we delve into the connection between cancer and diet, exploring the foods that are thought to have cancer-fighting potential.

Fruits and Vegetables: A diet rich in fruits and vegetables provides essential nutrients and antioxidants that help protect cells from damage. Cruciferous vegetables (like broccoli, cauliflower, and Brussels sprouts) are particularly noteworthy, as they contain compounds like sulforaphane that may have anti-cancer effects. Additionally, brightly coloured fruits such as berries, citrus fruits, and tomatoes are rich in vitamins, minerals, and antioxidants that support a healthy immune system.

Whole Grains: Whole grains like brown rice, quinoa, whole wheat, and oats contain fibre and other compounds that promote digestive health and may help lower the risk of certain cancers, such as colorectal cancer. They also have a lower glycemic index, which can help regulate blood sugar levels and insulin production, potentially reducing cancer risk.

Lean Proteins: Diets high in red and processed meats have been associated with an increased risk of cancer, particularly colorectal cancer. Opt for lean protein sources like poultry, fish, legumes, and plant-based proteins to reduce your cancer risk and promote overall health.

Healthy Fats: Include almonds, seeds, almonds and olive oil in your diet as sources of healthy fats. These fats provide essential fatty acids and antioxidants that support cellular health. Omega-3 fatty acids found in fatty fish like salmon and flaxseeds have anti-inflammatory properties that may help prevent cancer development.

Spices and Herbs: Turmeric, garlic, ginger, and green tea are among the many herbs and spices that contain bioactive compounds with potential anti-cancer effects. For example, curcumin, a compound in turmeric, has been studied for its ability to inhibit the growth of cancer cells and suppress inflammation.

Limit Processed Foods and Sugars: High intake of processed foods, sugary snacks, and sugary beverages can lead to obesity and insulin resistance, both of which are linked to an increased risk of cancer. Minimise your consumption of these foods and focus on whole, nutrient-dense options instead.

Hydration: Staying adequately hydrated is essential for overall health and may play a role in cancer prevention. Water helps with digestion, detoxification, and the maintenance of healthy cells.

INCORPORATING CANCER-FIGHTING FOODS INTO YOUR MEALS

While genetics and environmental factors play a role, a well-balanced diet rich in cancer-fighting foods can significantly contribute to reducing the risk of developing cancer and supporting overall health. Incorporating these foods into your meals is a proactive step toward promoting wellness. Here, we'll explore various foods that have been associated with cancer-fighting properties and provide tips on how to include them in your diet.

Colourful Fruits and Vegetables:
Vibrant fruits and vegetables are packed with antioxidants, vitamins, minerals, and fibre that help protect cells from damage and support a strong immune system. Aim for a variety of colours to ensure you're getting a wide range of nutrients. Examples include:

- Berries (blueberries, strawberries, raspberries)
- Cruciferous vegetables (broccoli, cauliflower, Brussels sprouts)
- Leafy greens (spinach, kale, Swiss chard)
- Citrus fruits (oranges, grapefruits, lemons)

Incorporation Tip:
Create colourful salads, smoothies, or stir-fries to combine multiple cancer-fighting ingredients in one meal.

Whole Grains:
Whole grains are rich in fibre, vitamins, and minerals that support digestion and reduce the risk of certain cancers, particularly colorectal cancer.

- Brown rice
- Quinoa
- Whole wheat
- Oats

Incorporation Tip:
Replace refined grains with whole grains in your meals, such as using whole wheat pasta or brown rice instead of their refined counterparts.

Lean Proteins:
Lean sources of protein provide the building blocks necessary for cell repair and immune function without excess saturated fat. Fish, poultry, beans, and legumes are excellent choices.

- Fatty fish (salmon, mackerel, sardines)
- Skinless poultry
- Lentils
- Chickpeas

Incorporation Tip:
Substitute red meat with lean protein sources in
dishes like salads, stews, or wraps.

Healthy Fats:
Certain fats, such as omega-3 fatty acids, have
anti-inflammatory properties that can help reduce the
risk of chronic diseases, including cancer.
- Avocado
- Nuts (walnuts, almonds, pistachios)
- Seeds (flaxseeds, chia seeds)

Incorporation Tip:
Add a handful of nuts or seeds to your breakfast
cereal or yoghourt for an extra dose of healthy fats.

Herbs and Spices:
Many herbs and spices contain potent compounds
that have been linked to cancer prevention and
suppression of tumour growth.
- Turmeric
- Garlic
- Ginger
- Rosemary

Incorporation Tip:
Incorporate these herbs and spices into your cooking
or make a flavorful marinade for grilled proteins.

It's important to note that while certain foods and
dietary patterns are associated with a lower risk of
cancer, there is no single "magic" food that can
prevent or cure cancer. A well-balanced diet rich in
nutrient-dense foods is essential. Additionally,
maintaining a healthy weight, engaging in regular

physical activity, avoiding tobacco and excessive alcohol consumption, and managing stress are all crucial components of a holistic approach to cancer prevention.

Before making significant dietary changes, it's advisable to consult with a healthcare professional, especially if you're undergoing cancer treatment or have specific dietary needs. They can provide personalised guidance based on your individual health status and goals.

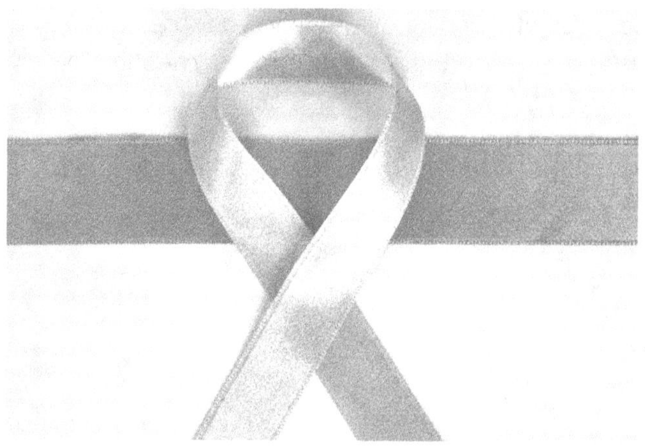

BREAKFAST RECIPES

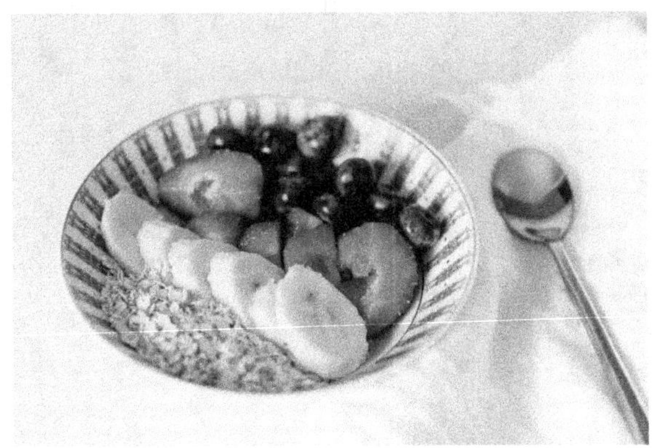

1. **Berry Oatmeal**:

Ingredients:

- 1/2 cup rolled oats
- 1 cup of almond milk (or any milk alternative)
- 1/2 cup mixed berries (blueberries, strawberries, raspberries)
- 1 tablespoon flax seeds
- 1 teaspoon honey or maple syrup (optional)

Instructions:

1. In a saucepan, combine oats and almond milk. Cook over a small amount of heat until the oats are tender and the mixture thickens.

2. Stir in mixed berries and flax seeds.

3. Cook for a few more minutes until the berries soften and release their juices.

4. Remove from heat, drizzle with honey or maple syrup if desired, and serve.

2. **Spinach and Mushroom Egg White Scramble**:

Ingredients:

- 3 egg whites
- 1 cup baby spinach leaves
- 1/2 cup sliced mushrooms
- 1/4 cup diced tomatoes
- 1 teaspoon olive oil
- Salt and pepper to taste

Instructions:

1. In a nonstick skillet over a small amount of heat, heat the olive oil.

2. Add sliced mushrooms and sauté until they start to brown.

3. Add baby spinach and diced tomatoes, cooking until the spinach wilts.

4. Pour in the egg whites and cook, stirring gently, until they are cooked through.

5. Season with salt and pepper, and serve.

3. **Greek Yoghourt Parfait**:

Ingredients:

- 1 cup Greek yoghourt
- 1/4 cup mixed nuts (walnuts, almonds, pistachios)
- 1/2 cup mixed fruits (berries, kiwi, pomegranate seeds)
- 1 tablespoon chia seeds
- 1 teaspoon honey

Instructions:

1. In a glass or bowl, layer Greek yogurt, mixed nuts, mixed fruits, and chia seeds.

2. Drizzle honey over top for extra sweetness.

3. Enjoy as a delicious and nutritious parfait.

4.

4. **Whole Grain Toast with Avocado and Salmon**:

Ingredients:

- 2 slices whole grain bread, toasted
- 1 ripe avocado, mashed
- 4 oz smoked salmon
- Sliced red onion
- Fresh dill
- Lemon juice
- Salt and pepper to taste

Instructions:

1. Spread mashed avocado evenly over the toasted bread slices.

2. Top with smoked salmon, sliced red onion, and fresh dill.

3. Season with salt and pepper after drizzling with lemon juice.

4. Serve open-faced for a satisfying breakfast.

5. **Turmeric Smoothie**:

Ingredients:

- 1 cup coconut milk (or any other preferred milk)
- 1 frozen banana
- 1/2 teaspoon turmeric powder
- 1/2 teaspoon ginger powder
- 1 tablespoon chia seeds
- 1 teaspoon honey

Instructions:

1. Blend coconut milk, frozen banana, turmeric powder, ginger powder, and chia seeds until smooth.

2. Sweeten with honey to taste.

3. Pour into a glass and enjoy the anti-inflammatory benefits of turmeric.

6. **Green Tea and Quinoa Bowl**:

Ingredients:

- 1 cup cooked quinoa
- 1 cup steamed broccoli florets
- 1 poached egg
- 1 teaspoon sesame seeds
- 1 cup green tea

Instructions:

1. In a bowl, assemble cooked quinoa and steamed broccoli.
2. Top with a poached egg and sprinkle sesame seeds over the top.
3. Enjoy with a cup of green tea, rich in antioxidants.

LUNCH RECIPES

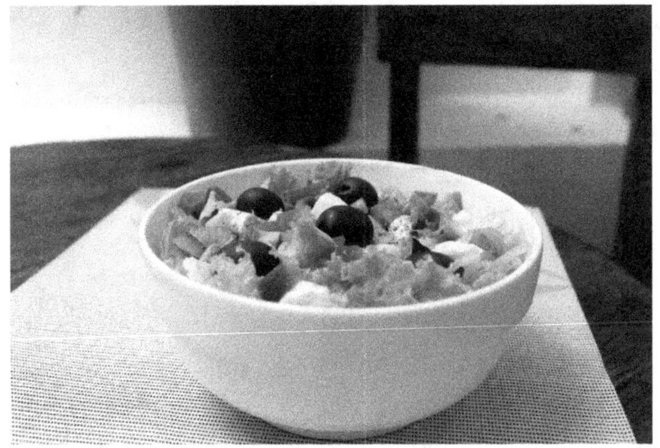

1. Spinach and Berry Salad:

Ingredients:
- Fresh spinach leaves
- Mixed berries (blueberries, strawberries, raspberries)
- Nuts (walnuts, almonds)
- Feta cheese (optional)
- Balsamic vinaigrette dressing

Instructions:
1. Dry after washing the berries and spinach leaves.
2. Toss the spinach, mixed berries, nuts, and feta cheese together in a bowl.
3. Drizzle with balsamic vinaigrette dressing just before serving.

2. **Turmeric Quinoa Bowl**:

Ingredients:
- Cooked quinoa
- Cooked black beans
- Steamed broccoli
- Diced carrots
- Turmeric powder
- Lemon juice
- Olive oil

Instructions:
1. In a bowl, combine cooked quinoa, black beans, steamed broccoli, and diced carrots.
2. Sprinkle turmeric powder over the bowl for its anti-inflammatory properties.
3. Drizzle with lemon juice and a touch of olive oil for flavour.

3. **Garlic Sautéed Greens**:

Ingredients:
- Assorted dark leafy greens (kale, Swiss chard, spinach)
- Garlic cloves (sliced)
- Lemon zest
- Crushed red pepper flakes (optional)
- Olive oil

Instructions:
1. Add sliced garlic after heating the olive oil in a pan. Sauté until fragrant.

2. Add the assorted greens and sauté until wilted.
3. Sprinkle lemon zest and crushed red pepper flakes for added flavour.

4. **Grilled Salmon Salad**:

Ingredients:
- Grilled salmon fillet
- Mixed salad greens
- Cherry tomatoes
- Sliced cucumber
- Avocado slices
- Pumpkin seeds
- Olive oil and lemon dressing

Instructions:
1. Place the grilled salmon fillet on a bed of mixed salad greens.
2. Arrange cherry tomatoes, sliced cucumber, avocado slices, and pumpkin seeds around the salmon.
3. Drizzle with a mixture of olive oil and lemon juice for dressing.

5. **Whole Grain Wrap with Hummus**:

Ingredients:
- Whole grain wrap or tortilla
- Hummus

- Grilled chicken slices (or roasted vegetables for a vegetarian option)
- Sliced bell peppers
- Shredded carrots
- Baby spinach leaves

Instructions:

1. Spread a generous layer of hummus onto the whole grain wrap.
2. Layer grilled chicken slices or roasted vegetables on top of the hummus.
3. Add sliced bell peppers, shredded carrots, and baby spinach leaves.
4. Roll up the wrap and enjoy.

6. **Lentil and Vegetable Soup**:

Ingredients:

- Cooked green or brown lentils
- Chopped mixed vegetables (carrots, celery, onion, zucchini)
- Low-sodium vegetable broth
- Turmeric and cumin spices
- Fresh parsley (chopped)
- Salt and pepper to taste

Instructions:

1. In a pot, sauté chopped vegetables until slightly softened.
2. Add cooked lentils, vegetable broth, turmeric, and cumin.
3. Simmer until the flavours meld together.
4. Season with salt, pepper, and chopped fresh parsley before serving.

DINNER RECIPES

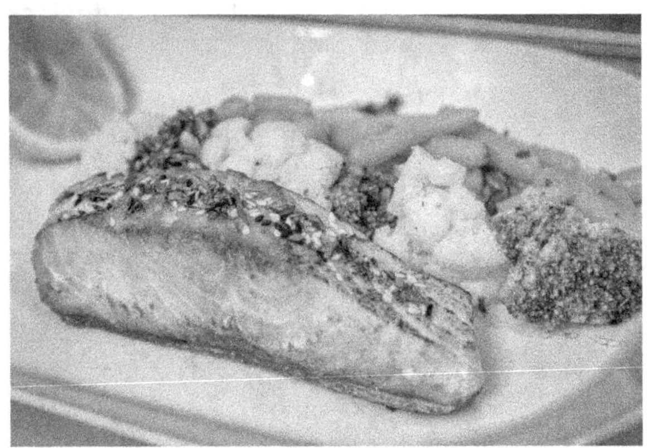

1. **Grilled Salmon with Broccoli and Turmeric Quinoa**:

Salmon is rich in omega-3 fatty acids, while broccoli and turmeric contain antioxidants and anti-inflammatory compounds.

Ingredients:
- 2 salmon fillets
- 2 cups broccoli florets
- 1 cup quinoa
- 2 teaspoons turmeric powder
- Salt and pepper to taste
- Olive oil

Instructions:
1. Cook quinoa according to package instructions, adding turmeric to the cooking water. Fluff with a fork when done.

2. Preheat the grill or oven. Season with salt and pepper after brushing salmon with olive oil.
3. Grill or bake salmon for about 4-5 minutes per side until cooked through.
4. Steam or blanch broccoli until tender.
5. Serve salmon over turmeric quinoa, with steamed broccoli on the side.

2. Tomato and Spinach Whole Wheat Pasta:

Tomatoes contain lycopene, a powerful antioxidant, and spinach is rich in vitamins and minerals.

Ingredients:
- Whole wheat pasta
- 2 cups fresh spinach
- 2 cups cherry tomatoes, halved
- 3 cloves garlic, minced
- 2 tablespoons olive oil
- Red pepper flakes (optional)
- Salt and pepper to taste
- Grated Parmesan cheese (optional)

Instructions:
1. Cook whole wheat pasta according to package instructions. Drain and set aside.
2. Heat olive oil over a small amount of heat in a large skillet. Add minced garlic and red pepper flakes, sauté for a minute.
3. Cook cherry tomatoes until they start to get soft after adding them.
4. Add spinach and cook until wilted.

5. Toss cooked pasta with the tomato and spinach mixture. Season with salt and pepper.
6. Top with grated Parmesan cheese if desired.

3. **Grilled Vegetable and Quinoa Stuffed Bell Peppers**:

Bell peppers are packed with vitamin C and antioxidants, while quinoa provides protein and fibre.

Ingredients:
- 3 bell peppers, halved and seeds removed
- 1 cup cooked quinoa
- 1 zucchini, diced
- 1 yellow squash, diced
- 1 red onion, diced
- 1 cup cherry tomatoes, halved
- 2 cloves garlic, minced
- 2 tablespoons olive oil
- 1 teaspoon dried herbs (such as thyme, oregano, or basil)
- Salt and pepper to taste

Instructions:
1. Preheat the grill or oven. Brush bell pepper halves with olive oil and grill/bake until slightly softened.
2. Heat olive oil over small amount of heat in a skillet. Add garlic and sauté until fragrant.
3. Add zucchini, yellow squash, and red onion. Cook until vegetables are tender.
4. Stir in cherry tomatoes and cooked quinoa. Season with dried herbs, salt, and pepper.

5. Stuff the grilled bell pepper halves with the vegetable-quinoa mixture.
6. Place the stuffed peppers back on the grill or in the oven for a few minutes to heat through.

4. **Garlic and Ginger Stir-Fry with Tofu**:

Garlic and ginger have anti-inflammatory properties, and tofu is a good source of plant-based protein.

Ingredients:
- 1 block firm tofu, cubed
- 2 cups mixed stir-fry vegetables (broccoli, carrots, bell peppers, snap peas, etc.)
- 3 cloves garlic, minced
- 1 tablespoon fresh ginger, minced
- 2 tablespoons soy sauce (low-sodium)
- 1 tablespoon sesame oil
- 1 tablespoon olive oil
- Red pepper flakes (optional)
- Brown rice or quinoa (for serving)

Instructions:
1. Cut the tofu into cubes after pressing to remove excess moisture.
2. In a bowl, whisk together soy sauce, sesame oil, and a pinch of red pepper flakes.
3. Heat olive oil in a wok or large skillet over medium to high amount of heat.
4. Sauté for a minute until fragrant after adding minced garlic.

5. Add tofu cubes and stir-fry until they start to brown.
6. Stir-fry the mixed vegetables until tender-crisp after adding them.
7. Pour the sauce over the tofu and vegetables, toss to coat.
8. Serve over brown rice or quinoa.

5. **Lentil and Vegetable Curry**:

Lentils are rich in protein and fibre, while turmeric and other spices in curry have anti-inflammatory properties.

Ingredients:

- 1 cup of dried brown or green lentils, drained after rinsing
- 1 onion, finely chopped
- 2 carrots, diced
- 1 red bell pepper, diced
- 1 cup cauliflower florets
- 2 cloves garlic, minced
- 1 tablespoon fresh ginger, minced
- 1 can (14 oz) diced tomatoes
- 1 can (14 oz) coconut milk (light)
- 2 tablespoons curry powder
- 1 teaspoon ground turmeric
- 1 teaspoon ground cumin
- 1 tablespoon olive oil
- Salt and pepper to taste
- Fresh cilantro, chopped (for garnish)
- Cooked brown rice (for serving)

Instructions:

1. Heat olive oil over a small amount of heat in a large pot. Add chopped onion, garlic, and ginger. Sauté until onion is translucent.
2. Add curry powder, ground turmeric, and ground cumin. Also cook for a while to toast the spices.
3. Add diced tomatoes, coconut milk, lentils, and vegetables. Season with salt and pepper.
4. Bring to a boil, then reduce heat, cover, and simmer until lentils are tender or for about 25-30 minutes.
5. Serve the lentil curry over cooked brown rice, garnished with fresh cilantro.

6. **Roasted Garlic and Spinach Stuffed Mushrooms**:

Garlic and spinach are rich in antioxidants, and mushrooms are a good source of nutrients.

Ingredients:
- Large mushroom caps (portobello or cremini)
- 2 cups fresh spinach, chopped
- 1 head garlic
- 2 tablespoons olive oil
- ¼ cup breadcrumbs (whole wheat)
- ¼ cup grated Parmesan cheese
- Salt and pepper to taste

Instructions:
1. Preheat the oven to 400°F (200°C).
2. Cut the top off the garlic head to expose the cloves. Drizzle with olive oil, wrap in

aluminium foil, and roast for about 30 minutes
or until soft. Press to squeeze the roasted
garlic out of the cloves.
3. Remove stems from mushroom caps and
    gently scoop out some of the inner flesh to
    create space for the filling.
4. Heat olive oil over a small amount of heat in a
    skillet. Add chopped spinach and sauté until
    wilted.
5. In a bowl, combine the roasted garlic, sautéed
    spinach, breadcrumbs, and grated Parmesan.
    Season with salt and pepper.
6. Stuff each mushroom cap with the
    garlic-spinach mixture.
7. Place stuffed mushrooms on a baking sheet
    and bake for about 15-20 minutes, until
    mushrooms are tender and the filling is
    golden.

Remember that these recipes incorporate ingredients
that are believed to have cancer-fighting properties,
but they should be part of an overall balanced diet
and healthy lifestyle. It's essential to consult with a
healthcare professional for personalised advice and
recommendations, especially if you have specific
dictary restrictions or health concerns.

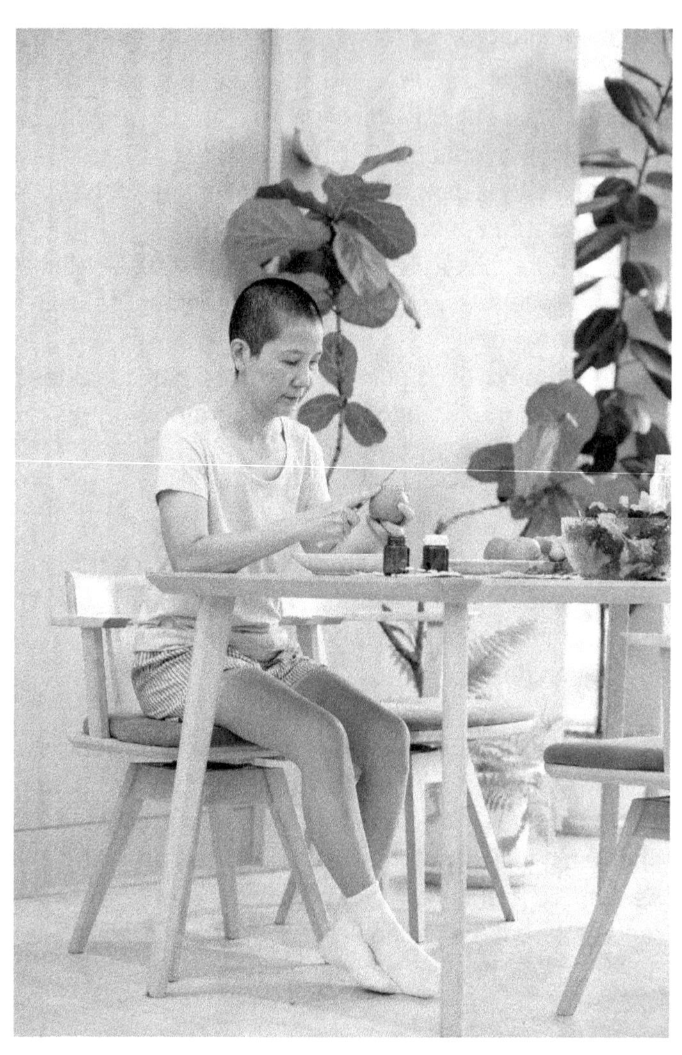

DESSERT RECIPES

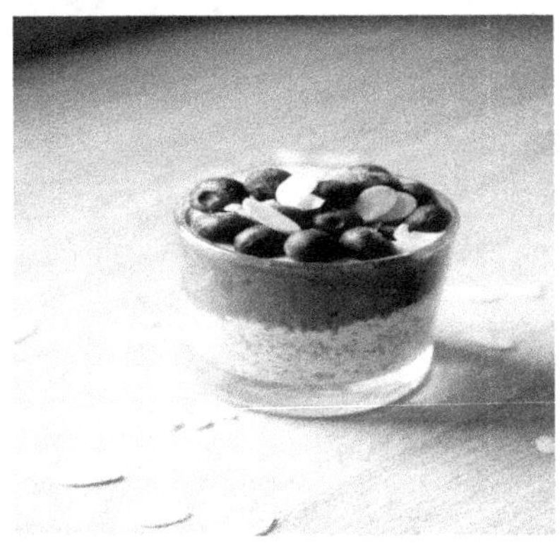

1. Blueberry Chia Seed Pudding:

Ingredients:
- 1 cup fresh blueberries
- 2 tbsp chia seeds
- 1 cup of almond milk (or any milk alternative)
- 1 tsp honey (optional)
- 1/2 tsp vanilla extract

Instructions:
1. Blend half of the blueberries with almond milk and honey (if using).
2. In a bowl, combine the blended mixture, chia seeds, and vanilla extract. Mix well.
3. Refrigerate for at least 2 hours or until the mixture thickens.
4. Serve the chia pudding topped with the remaining fresh blueberries.

2. **Dark Chocolate Avocado Mousse**:

Ingredients:
- 2 ripe avocados
- 1/4 cup cocoa powder (unsweetened)
- 1/4 cup honey or maple syrup
- 1 tsp vanilla extract
- A pinch of salt
- Fresh berries, for garnish

Instructions:
1. Scoop the flesh of avocados into a food processor.
2. Add cocoa powder, honey or maple syrup, vanilla extract, and a pinch of salt.
3. Blend until smooth and creamy.
4. Divide the mousse into serving dishes and refrigerate for about 1 hour.
5. Garnish with fresh berries before serving.

3. **Berry-Oat Crumble Bars**:

Ingredients:
- 1 cup rolled oats
- 1/2 cup whole wheat flour
- 1/4 cup coconut oil
- 1/4 cup honey or maple syrup
- 2 cups mixed berries (e.g., raspberries, strawberries, blackberries)
- 1 tsp lemon juice
- 1 tsp grated lemon zest

Instructions:
1. Preheat the oven to 350°F (175°C) and line a baking dish with parchment paper.

2. In a bowl, combine oats, whole wheat flour, melted coconut oil, and honey or maple syrup to make the crumble mixture.
3. Press two-thirds of the crumble mixture into the bottom of the baking dish to form the base.
4. In another bowl, mix the berries with lemon juice and zest.
5. Spread the berry mixture over the crumble base.
6. Sprinkle the remaining crumble mixture on top of the berries.
7. Bake until the top is golden brown or for 25-30 minutes.
8. Allow to cool before cutting into bars.

4. **Turmeric Mango Sorbet**:

Ingredients:
- 2 ripe mangoes, peeled and diced
- 1 tsp turmeric powder
- 1 tbsp fresh ginger, grated
- 2 tbsp honey or agave nectar
- Juice of 1 lime

Instructions:
1. Blend the diced mangoes, turmeric, ginger, honey or agave nectar, and lime juice until smooth.
2. Pour the mixture into a freezer-safe container.
3. Freeze for about 4 hours, stirring every hour to prevent ice crystals from forming.
4. Serve the sorbet with a sprinkle of turmeric on top.

5. **Walnut-Date Energy Bites**:

Ingredients:
- 1 cup walnuts
- 1 cup pitted dates
- 2 tbsp unsweetened cocoa powder
- 1 tsp vanilla extract
- A pinch of salt
- Desiccated coconut (for rolling)

Instructions:
1. In a food processor, blend walnuts, dates, cocoa powder, vanilla extract, and salt until a sticky mixture forms.
2. Roll the mixture into small bite-sized balls.
3. Roll each ball in desiccated coconut to coat.
4. Refrigerate for about 1 hour before serving.

6. **Pomegranate Yoghourt Parfait**:

Ingredients:
- 1 cup Greek yoghourt
- 1/2 cup pomegranate seeds
- 1/4 cup granola (preferably with nuts)
- 1 tbsp honey
- 1 tsp ground flaxseed

Instructions:
1. In serving glasses, layer Greek yoghourt, pomegranate seeds, and granola.
2. Drizzle honey over each layer.
3. Until the glasses are filled, keep repeating the layers.
4. Top with a sprinkle of ground flaxseed before serving.

SNACKS AND APPETISERS

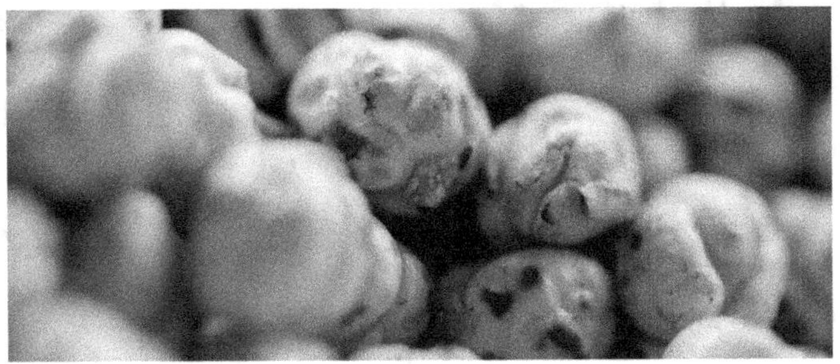

1. Turmeric Roasted Chickpeas:

Ingredients:
- 1 can of chickpeas(15 oz), rinsed and drained
- 1 tablespoon olive oil
- 1 teaspoon ground turmeric
- 1/2 teaspoon ground cumin
- 1/2 teaspoon paprika
- Salt and pepper to taste

Instructions:
1. Preheat the oven to 400°F (200°C).
2. In a bowl, toss the chickpeas with olive oil, turmeric, cumin, paprika, salt, and pepper until well coated.
3. On a baking sheet in a single layer spread the chickpeas.
4. Roast in the oven until crispy and golden brown or for 20-25 minutes.
5. Allow to cool before serving as a crunchy and flavorful snack.

2. **Spinach and Kale Stuffed Mushrooms**:

Ingredients:
- 12 large button mushrooms, stems removed
- 1 cup baby spinach, chopped
- 1 cup kale, de stemmed and chopped
- 1/4 cup finely chopped onion
- 2 cloves garlic, minced
- 1/4 cup grated Parmesan cheese
- Salt and pepper to taste

Instructions:
1. Preheat the oven to 375°F (190°C).
2. Sauté the onion and garlic until they are softened in a skillet.
3. Add the chopped spinach and kale, and cook until wilted.
4. Stir in the Parmesan cheese and season with salt and pepper.
5. Fill each mushroom cap with the spinach-kale mixture.
6. Place the stuffed mushrooms on a baking sheet and bake for 15-20 minutes, until mushrooms are tender.

3. **Rainbow Vegetable Skewers**:

Ingredients:
- Cherry tomatoes
- Red bell pepper, cut into chunks
- Yellow bell pepper, cut into chunks
- Green zucchini, sliced
- Purple onion, cut into chunks

- Mushrooms, cleaned and halved
- Olive oil
- Fresh herbs (such as rosemary or thyme)
- Salt and pepper to taste

Instructions:

1. Over a small amount of heat, preheat the grill or grill pan..Thread the vegetables onto skewers, alternating colours.
2. Brush the skewers with olive oil and sprinkle with fresh herbs, salt, and pepper.
3. Grill the skewers for about 10-15 minutes, turning occasionally, until vegetables are charred and tender.
4. Serve the rainbow vegetable skewers as colourful and nutritious appetisers.

4. **Citrusy Quinoa Salad Cups**:

Ingredients:

- Mini phyllo dough cups
- 1 cup cooked quinoa, cooled
- Orange segments, chopped
- Cucumber, diced
- Red onion, finely chopped
- Chopped fresh mint and parsley
- Juice of 1 lemon
- Olive oil
- Salt and pepper to taste

Instructions:

1. In a bowl, combine the cooked quinoa, orange segments, cucumber, red onion, mint, and parsley.

2. Drizzle with lemon juice and olive oil.Toss to combine after seasoning with salt and pepper.
3. Spoon the quinoa salad into mini phyllo dough cups.
4. Chill in the refrigerator for a bit before serving, allowing the flavours to meld.

5. **Almond Butter and Berry Rice Cakes**:

Ingredients:
- Rice cakes
- Almond butter
- Mixed berries (such as blueberries, raspberries, and strawberries)
- Chia seeds

Instructions:
1. Spread almond butter on each rice cake.
2. Top with a variety of mixed berries.
3. Sprinkle chia seeds over the berries for added crunch and nutrients.
4. These rice cake snacks are quick to assemble and packed with antioxidants.

6. **Greek Yogurt and Veggie Dip**:

Ingredients:
- 1 cup Greek yoghourt
- 1/2 cup of grated cucumber, pressed to remove excess moisture
- 1 clove garlic, minced
- 1 tablespoon chopped fresh dill
- 1 tablespoon lemon juice
- Salt and pepper to taste

Instructions:
1. In a bowl, combine Greek yoghourt, grated cucumber, minced garlic, dill, and lemon juice.
2. Mix well after seasoning with salt and pepper.
3. Chill the dip in the refrigerator for at least 30 minutes to let the flavours meld.
4. Serve with an assortment of fresh vegetables like carrot sticks, sliced cucumbers, and stripped bell peppers.

Remember to enjoy these snacks and appetisers as part of a well-balanced diet. While certain foods have shown potential cancer-fighting properties, maintaining a healthy lifestyle, avoiding tobacco and excessive alcohol consumption, staying physically active, and regular screenings are also crucial for cancer prevention.

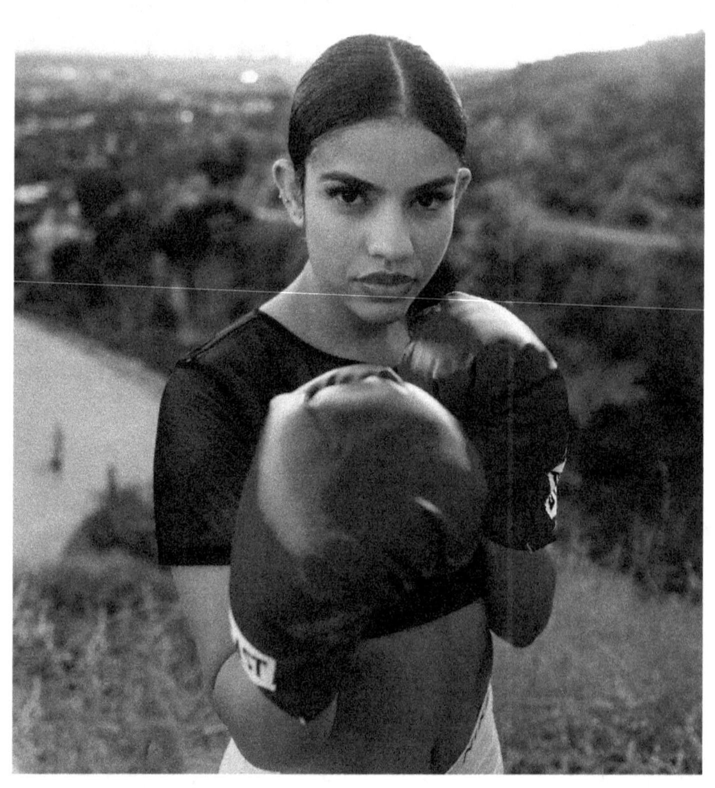

Conclusion

In conclusion, the "Foods That Beat Cancer Cookbook" serves as an invaluable resource for both cancer prevention and those who have been newly diagnosed. This cookbook goes beyond being a mere collection of recipes; it stands as a testament to the empowering role that nutrition can play in the battle against cancer.

For those seeking to prevent cancer, this cookbook offers a comprehensive guide to incorporating cancer-fighting foods into their daily lives. By emphasising a diverse range of fruits, vegetables, whole grains, lean proteins, and antioxidants, the cookbook provides practical and delicious ways to strengthen the body's defences against cancer development.

Equally important, for individuals who are facing a new cancer diagnosis, this cookbook provides not only nourishment but also hope and empowerment. The carefully crafted recipes take into consideration the unique nutritional needs that may arise during cancer treatment. From managing side effects to supporting the body's healing process, the cookbook equips patients with the tools to make informed dietary choices that can enhance their overall well-being.

Ultimately, the "Foods That Beat Cancer Cookbook" underscores the profound connection between food and health. It encourages a proactive approach to wellness through the choices we make at the dinner table. By embracing the principles outlined in this cookbook, individuals can embark on a journey towards better health, armed with knowledge, resilience, and a renewed sense of control. As research continues to illuminate the intricate relationship between nutrition and cancer, this cookbook stands as a beacon of practicality and optimism, offering a path to a healthier and more vibrant life.

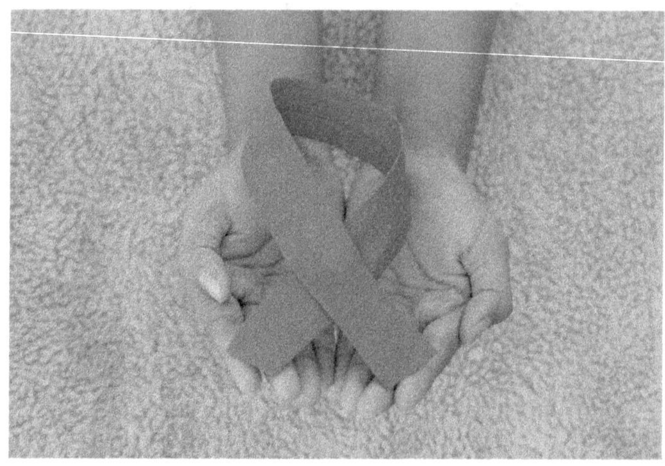

REVIEW